180-Day
Food Tracker
(Track What You Eat)

Created by: Trueheart Designs

Today's Date: | No. of Calories

Breakfast:

_____

_____

_____

_____

_____

_____

_____

_____

Lunch:

_____

_____

_____

_____

_____

_____

	No. of Calories
Dinner:	
Snacks & Beverages (including Water) :	
	Grand Total:

Today's Date: No. of Calories

Breakfast:

Lunch:

	No. of Calories
Dinner:	
Snacks & Beverages (including Water) :	
	Grand Total:

Today's Date: | No. of Calories

Breakfast:

_____

_____

_____

_____

_____

_____

_____

_____

Lunch:

_____

_____

_____

_____

_____

_____

_____

	No. of Calories
Dinner:	
Snacks & Beverages (including Water) :	
	Grand Total:

Today's Date: | No. of Calories

Breakfast:

_____

_____

_____

_____

_____

_____

_____

_____

Lunch:

_____

_____

_____

_____

_____

_____

_____

_____

No. of Calories

Dinner:

Snacks & Beverages (including Water) :

Grand Total:

Today's Date:	No. of Calories
Breakfast:	
Lunch:	

	No. of Calories
Dinner:	
Snacks & Beverages (including Water) :	
	Grand Total:

Today's Date: | No. of Calories

Breakfast:

_____

_____

_____

_____

_____

_____

_____

_____

Lunch:

_____

_____

_____

_____

_____

_____

_____

No. of Calories

Dinner:

_____

_____

_____

_____

_____

_____

_____

Snacks & Beverages (including Water) :

_____

_____

_____

_____

_____

_____

Grand Total:

_____

_____

Today's Date: | No. of Calories

Breakfast:

Lunch:

	No. of Calories
Dinner:	
Snacks & Beverages (including Water) :	
	Grand Total:

Today's Date:	No. of Calories
Breakfast:	
Lunch:	

	No. of Calories
Dinner:	
Snacks & Beverages (including Water) :	
	Grand Total:

Today's Date: | No. of Calories

Breakfast:

_____

_____

_____

_____

_____

_____

_____

_____

Lunch:

_____

_____

_____

_____

_____

_____

_____

	No. of Calories
Dinner:	
Snacks & Beverages (including Water) :	
	Grand Total:

Today's Date: | No. of Calories

Breakfast:

_____

Lunch:

	No. of Calories
Dinner:	
Snacks & Beverages (including Water) :	
	Grand Total:

Today's Date: No. of Calories

Breakfast:

Lunch:

	No. of Calories
Dinner:	
Snacks & Beverages (including Water) :	
	Grand Total:

Today's Date:	No. of Calories
Breakfast:

Lunch:

	No. of Calories
Dinner:	
Snacks & Beverages (including Water) :	
	Grand Total:

Today's Date: | No. of Calories

Breakfast:

Lunch:

	No. of Calories
Dinner:	
Snacks & Beverages (including Water) :	
	Grand Total:

Today's Date: | No. of Calories

Breakfast:

Lunch:

	No. of Calories
Dinner:	
Snacks & Beverages (including Water) :	
	Grand Total:

Today's Date: _____ | No. of Calories

Breakfast: _____ | _____

_____ | _____

_____ | _____

_____ | _____

_____ | _____

_____ | _____

_____ | _____

_____ | _____

_____ | _____

Lunch: _____ | _____

_____ | _____

_____ | _____

_____ | _____

_____ | _____

_____ | _____

_____ | _____

_____ | _____

_____ | _____

	No. of Calories
Dinner:	
Snacks & Beverages (including Water) :	
	Grand Total:

Today's Date: No. of Calories

Breakfast:

Lunch:

	No. of Calories
Dinner:	
Snacks & Beverages (including Water):	
	Grand Total:

Today's Date:	No. of Calories
Breakfast:	
Lunch:	

	No. of Calories
Dinner:	
Snacks & Beverages (including Water) :	
	Grand Total:

Today's Date: | No. of Calories

Breakfast:

Lunch:

	No. of Calories
Dinner:	
Snacks & Beverages (including Water) :	
	Grand Total:

Today's Date: | No. of Calories

Breakfast:

Lunch:

	No. of Calories
Dinner:	
Snacks & Beverages (including Water) :	
	Grand Total:

Today's Date: | No. of Calories

Breakfast:

Lunch:

	No. of Calories
Dinner:	
Snacks & Beverages (including Water) :	
	Grand Total:

Today's Date:	No. of Calories
Breakfast:	
Lunch:	

	No. of Calories
Dinner:	
Snacks & Beverages (including Water) :	
	Grand Total:

Today's Date: | No. of Calories

Breakfast:

Lunch:

	No. of Calories
Dinner:	
Snacks & Beverages (including Water) :	
	Grand Total:

Today's Date: | No. of Calories

Breakfast:

_____

_____

_____

_____

_____

_____

_____

_____

Lunch:

_____

_____

_____

_____

_____

_____

_____

_____

	No. of Calories
Dinner:	
Snacks & Beverages (including Water) :	
	Grand Total:

Today's Date: | No. of Calories

Breakfast:

Lunch:

	No. of Calories
Dinner:	
Snacks & Beverages (including Water) :	
	Grand Total:

Today's Date:	No. of Calories
Breakfast:	
Lunch:	

	No. of Calories
Dinner:	
Snacks & Beverages (including Water) :	
	Grand Total:

Today's Date: | No. of Calories

Breakfast:

Lunch:

	No. of Calories
Dinner:	
Snacks & Beverages (including Water) :	
	Grand Total:

Today's Date: | No. of Calories

Breakfast:

Lunch:

	No. of Calories
Dinner:	
Snacks & Beverages (including Water) :	
	Grand Total:

Today's Date: | No. of Calories

Breakfast:

Lunch:

	No. of Calories
Dinner:	
Snacks & Beverages (including Water) :	
	Grand Total:

Today's Date:	No. of Calories
Breakfast:	
Lunch:	

	No. of Calories
Dinner:	
Snacks & Beverages (including Water) :	
	Grand Total:

Today's Date: No. of Calories

Breakfast:

_____

_____

_____

_____

_____

_____

_____

_____

Lunch:

_____

_____

_____

_____

_____

_____

_____

	No. of Calories
Dinner:	
Snacks & Beverages (including Water) :	
	Grand Total:

Today's Date: | No. of Calories

Breakfast:

Lunch:

	No. of Calories
Dinner:	
Snacks & Beverages (including Water) :	
	Grand Total:

Today's Date: | No. of Calories

Breakfast:

Lunch:

	No. of Calories
Dinner:	
Snacks & Beverages (including Water) :	
	Grand Total:

Today's Date:	No. of Calories
Breakfast:	
Lunch:	

	No. of Calories
Dinner:	
Snacks & Beverages (including Water) :	
	Grand Total:

Today's Date: | No. of Calories

Breakfast:

Lunch:

	No. of Calories
Dinner:	
Snacks & Beverages (including Water):	
	Grand Total:

Today's Date: | No. of Calories

Breakfast:

_____

_____

_____

_____

_____

_____

_____

_____

Lunch:

_____

_____

_____

_____

_____

_____

_____

_____

	No. of Calories
Dinner:	
Snacks & Beverages (including Water) :	
	Grand Total:

Today's Date: | No. of Calories

Breakfast:

Lunch:

	No. of Calories
Dinner:	
Snacks & Beverages (including Water):	
	Grand Total:

Today's Date:	No. of Calories
Breakfast:	
Lunch:	

	No. of Calories
Dinner:	
Snacks & Beverages (including Water) :	
	Grand Total:

Today's Date: No. of Calories

Breakfast:

Lunch:

	No. of Calories
Dinner:	
Snacks & Beverages (including Water) :	
	Grand Total:

Today's Date: | No. of Calories

Breakfast:

Lunch:

	No. of Calories
Dinner:	
Snacks & Beverages (including Water) :	
	Grand Total:

Today's Date: | No. of Calories

Breakfast:

Lunch:

	No. of Calories
Dinner:	
Snacks & Beverages (including Water) :	
	Grand Total:

Today's Date: | No. of Calories

Breakfast:

Lunch:

No. of Calories

Dinner:

_____

_____

_____

_____

_____

_____

_____

_____

Snacks & Beverages (including Water):

_____

_____

_____

_____

_____

_____

Grand Total:

_____

Today's Date: | No. of Calories

Breakfast:

Lunch:

	No. of Calories
Dinner:	
Snacks & Beverages (including Water) :	
	Grand Total:

Today's Date:	No. of Calories
Breakfast:	
Lunch:	

	No. of Calories
Dinner:	
Snacks & Beverages (including Water) :	
	Grand Total:

Today's Date: | No. of Calories

Breakfast:

Lunch:

	No. of Calories
Dinner:	
Snacks & Beverages (including Water) :	
	Grand Total:

Today's Date: | No. of Calories

Breakfast:

Lunch:

	No. of Calories
Dinner:	
Snacks & Beverages (including Water):	
	Grand Total:

Today's Date: | No. of Calories

Breakfast:

Lunch:

	No. of Calories
Dinner:	
Snacks & Beverages (including Water) :	
	Grand Total:

Today's Date:	No. of Calories
Breakfast:	
Lunch:	

	No. of Calories
Dinner:	
Snacks & Beverages (including Water) :	
	Grand Total:

Today's Date: | No. of Calories

Breakfast:

_____

_____

_____

_____

_____

_____

_____

_____

Lunch:

_____

_____

_____

_____

_____

_____

_____

	No. of Calories
Dinner:	
Snacks & Beverages (including Water) :	
	Grand Total:

Today's Date: _____ | No. of Calories

Breakfast:

_____

_____

_____

_____

_____

_____

_____

_____

Lunch:

_____

_____

_____

_____

_____

_____

_____

	No. of Calories
Dinner:	
Snacks & Beverages (including Water):	
	Grand Total:

Today's Date: | No. of Calories

Breakfast:

Lunch:

	No. of Calories
Dinner:	
Snacks & Beverages (including Water) :	
	Grand Total:

Today's Date: | No. of Calories

Breakfast:

Lunch:

	No. of Calories
Dinner:	
Snacks & Beverages (including Water) :	
	Grand Total:

Today's Date: No. of Calories

Breakfast:

_____

_____

_____

_____

_____

_____

_____

_____

Lunch:

_____

_____

_____

_____

_____

_____

_____

	No. of Calories
Dinner:	
Snacks & Beverages (including Water):	
	Grand Total:

Today's Date: | No. of Calories

Breakfast:

Lunch:

	No. of Calories
Dinner:	
Snacks & Beverages (including Water) :	
	Grand Total:

Today's Date: | No. of Calories

Breakfast:

Lunch:

	No. of Calories
Dinner:	
Snacks & Beverages (including Water) :	
	Grand Total:

Today's Date:	No. of Calories
Breakfast:	
Lunch:	

	No. of Calories
Dinner:	
Snacks & Beverages (including Water) :	
	Grand Total:

Today's Date: | No. of Calories

Breakfast:

Lunch:

	No. of Calories
Dinner:	
Snacks & Beverages (including Water) :	
	Grand Total:

Today's Date: | No. of Calories

Breakfast:

Lunch:

	No. of Calories
Dinner:	
Snacks & Beverages (including Water) :	
	Grand Total:

Today's Date: | No. of Calories

Breakfast:

Lunch:

	No. of Calories
Dinner:	
Snacks & Beverages (including Water) :	
	Grand Total:

Today's Date: | No. of Calories

Breakfast:

_____

_____

_____

_____

_____

_____

_____

_____

Lunch:

_____

_____

_____

_____

_____

_____

_____

_____

	No. of Calories
Dinner:	
Snacks & Beverages (including Water) :	
	Grand Total:

Today's Date: | No. of Calories

Breakfast:

Lunch:

	No. of Calories
Dinner:	
Snacks & Beverages (including Water) :	
	Grand Total:

Today's Date: | No. of Calories

Breakfast:

Lunch:

	No. of Calories
Dinner:	
Snacks & Beverages (including Water) :	
	Grand Total:

Today's Date: | No. of Calories

Breakfast:

Lunch:

	No. of Calories
Dinner:	
Snacks & Beverages (including Water) :	
	Grand Total:

Today's Date:	No. of Calories
Breakfast:	
Lunch:	

No. of Calories

Dinner:

Snacks & Beverages (including Water) :

Grand Total:

Today's Date: No. of Calories

Breakfast:

Lunch:

	No. of Calories
Dinner:	
Snacks & Beverages (including Water) :	
	Grand Total:

Today's Date:	No. of Calories
Breakfast:	
Lunch:	

	No. of Calories
Dinner:	
Snacks & Beverages (including Water):	
	Grand Total:

Today's Date: No. of Calories

Breakfast:

_____ | _____

_____ | _____

_____ | _____

_____ | _____

_____ | _____

_____ | _____

_____ | _____

_____ | _____

Lunch:

_____ | _____

_____ | _____

_____ | _____

_____ | _____

_____ | _____

_____ | _____

_____ | _____

_____ | _____

	No. of Calories
Dinner:	
Snacks & Beverages (including Water) :	
	Grand Total:

Today's Date:	No. of Calories
Breakfast:	
Lunch:	

No. of Calories

Dinner:

Snacks & Beverages (including Water) :

Grand Total:

Today's Date: | No. of Calories

Breakfast:

_____

_____

_____

_____

_____

_____

_____

_____

Lunch:

_____

_____

_____

_____

_____

_____

_____

	No. of Calories
Dinner:	
Snacks & Beverages (including Water) :	
	Grand Total:

Today's Date:	No. of Calories
Breakfast:	
Lunch:	

	No. of Calories
Dinner:	
Snacks & Beverages (including Water) :	
	Grand Total:

Today's Date: | No. of Calories

Breakfast:

Lunch:

	No. of Calories
Dinner:	
Snacks & Beverages (including Water) :	
	Grand Total:

Today's Date:	No. of Calories
Breakfast:	
Lunch:	

	No. of Calories
Dinner:	
Snacks & Beverages (including Water) :	
	Grand Total:

Today's Date: | No. of Calories

Breakfast:

Lunch:

No. of Calories

Dinner:

Snacks & Beverages (including Water) :

Grand Total:

Today's Date: _____ | No. of Calories

Breakfast: _____

_____

_____

_____

_____

_____

_____

_____

Lunch: _____

_____

_____

_____

_____

_____

_____

_____

No. of Calories

Dinner:

Snacks & Beverages (including Water) :

Grand Total:

Today's Date: | No. of Calories

Breakfast:

Lunch:

No. of Calories

Dinner:

Snacks & Beverages (including Water) :

Grand Total:

Today's Date: | No. of Calories

Breakfast:

Lunch:

No. of Calories

Dinner:

Snacks & Beverages (including Water) :

Grand Total:

Today's Date: | No. of Calories

Breakfast:

Lunch:

	No. of Calories
Dinner:	
Snacks & Beverages (including Water) :	
	Grand Total:

Today's Date:	No. of Calories
Breakfast:	
Lunch:	

	No. of Calories
Dinner:	
Snacks & Beverages (including Water) :	
	Grand Total:

Today's Date: | No. of Calories

Breakfast:

_____

_____

_____

_____

_____

_____

_____

_____

Lunch:

_____

_____

_____

_____

_____

_____

_____

_____

	No. of Calories
Dinner:	
Snacks & Beverages (including Water) :	
	Grand Total:

Today's Date:	No. of Calories
Breakfast:	
Lunch:	

	No. of Calories
Dinner:	
Snacks & Beverages (including Water) :	
	Grand Total:

Today's Date: | No. of Calories

Breakfast:

Lunch:

	No. of Calories
Dinner:	
Snacks & Beverages (including Water) :	
	Grand Total:

Today's Date: | No. of Calories

Breakfast:

_____

_____

_____

_____

_____

_____

_____

_____

Lunch:

_____

_____

_____

_____

_____

_____

_____

_____

No. of Calories

Dinner:

Snacks & Beverages (including Water) :

Grand Total:

Today's Date:	No. of Calories
Breakfast:	
Lunch:	

	No. of Calories
Dinner:	
Snacks & Beverages (including Water) :	
	Grand Total:

Today's Date:	No. of Calories
Breakfast:	
Lunch:	

No. of Calories

Dinner:

Snacks & Beverages (including Water) :

Grand Total:

Today's Date: | No. of Calories

Breakfast:

Lunch:

	No. of Calories
Dinner:	
Snacks & Beverages (including Water) :	
	Grand Total:

Today's Date: | No. of Calories

Breakfast:

Lunch:

	No. of Calories
Dinner:	
Snacks & Beverages (including Water) :	
	Grand Total:

Today's Date: | No. of Calories

Breakfast:

Lunch:

	No. of Calories
Dinner:	
Snacks & Beverages (including Water) :	
	Grand Total:

Today's Date: | No. of Calories

Breakfast:

Lunch:

	No. of Calories
Dinner:	
Snacks & Beverages (including Water) :	
	Grand Total:

Today's Date: | No. of Calories

Breakfast:

_____

_____

_____

_____

_____

_____

_____

_____

Lunch:

_____

_____

_____

_____

_____

_____

_____

_____

No. of Calories

Dinner:

Snacks & Beverages (including Water) :

Grand Total:

Today's Date: | No. of Calories

Breakfast:

Lunch:

	No. of Calories
Dinner:	
Snacks & Beverages (including Water) :	
	Grand Total:

Today's Date: No. of Calories

Breakfast:

Lunch:

	No. of Calories
Dinner:	
Snacks & Beverages (including Water) :	
	Grand Total:

Today's Date: | No. of Calories

Breakfast:

_____

Lunch:

	No. of Calories
Dinner:	
Snacks & Beverages (including Water) :	
	Grand Total:

Today's Date: | No. of Calories

Breakfast:

Lunch:

	No. of Calories
Dinner:	
Snacks & Beverages (including Water) :	
	Grand Total:

Today's Date:	No. of Calories
Breakfast:	
Lunch:	

	No. of Calories
Dinner:	
Snacks & Beverages (including Water) :	
	Grand Total:

Today's Date: | No. of Calories

Breakfast:

_____

_____

_____

_____

_____

_____

_____

_____

Lunch:

_____

_____

_____

_____

_____

_____

_____

	No. of Calories
Dinner:	
Snacks & Beverages (including Water) :	
	Grand Total:

Today's Date:	No. of Calories
Breakfast:	
Lunch:	

	No. of Calories
Dinner:	
Snacks & Beverages (including Water) :	
	Grand Total:

Today's Date:	No. of Calories
Breakfast:	
Lunch:	

	No. of Calories
Dinner:	
Snacks & Beverages (including Water) :	
	Grand Total:

Today's Date: | No. of Calories

Breakfast:

Lunch:

	No. of Calories
Dinner:	
Snacks & Beverages (including Water) :	
	Grand Total:

Today's Date: No. of Calories

Breakfast:

Lunch:

No. of Calories

Dinner:

Snacks & Beverages (including Water) :

Grand Total:

Today's Date:	No. of Calories
Breakfast:	
Lunch:	

	No. of Calories
Dinner:	
Snacks & Beverages (including Water):	
	Grand Total:

Today's Date: No. of Calories

Breakfast:

Lunch:

	No. of Calories
Dinner:	
Snacks & Beverages (including Water) :	
	Grand Total:

Today's Date:	No. of Calories
Breakfast:	
Lunch:	

	No. of Calories
Dinner:	
Snacks & Beverages (including Water):	
	Grand Total:

Today's Date: | No. of Calories

Breakfast:

Lunch:

	No. of Calories
Dinner:	
Snacks & Beverages (including Water) :	
	Grand Total:

Today's Date: | No. of Calories

Breakfast:

Lunch:

	No. of Calories
Dinner:	
Snacks & Beverages (including Water) :	
	Grand Total:

Today's Date: | No. of Calories

Breakfast:

_____

Lunch:

	No. of Calories
Dinner:	
Snacks & Beverages (including Water) :	
	Grand Total:

Today's Date: No. of Calories

Breakfast:

Lunch:

No. of Calories

Dinner:

Snacks & Beverages (including Water):

Grand Total:

Today's Date: | No. of Calories

Breakfast:

Lunch:

	No. of Calories
Dinner:	
Snacks & Beverages (including Water) :	
	Grand Total:

Today's Date:	No. of Calories
Breakfast:	
Lunch:	

	No. of Calories
Dinner:	
Snacks & Beverages (including Water) :	
	Grand Total:

Today's Date:	No. of Calories
Breakfast:	
Lunch:	

	No. of Calories
Dinner:	
Snacks & Beverages (including Water) :	
	Grand Total:

Today's Date: | No. of Calories

Breakfast:

Lunch:

	No. of Calories
Dinner:	
Snacks & Beverages (including Water) :	
	Grand Total:

Today's Date: No. of Calories

Breakfast:

Lunch:

	No. of Calories
Dinner:	
Snacks & Beverages (including Water) :	
	Grand Total:

Today's Date:	No. of Calories
Breakfast:	
Lunch:	

	No. of Calories
Dinner:	
Snacks & Beverages (including Water) :	
	Grand Total:

Today's Date: | No. of Calories

Breakfast:

Lunch:

	No. of Calories
Dinner:	
Snacks & Beverages (including Water) :	
	Grand Total:

Today's Date:	No. of Calories
Breakfast:	
Lunch:	

	No. of Calories
Dinner:	
Snacks & Beverages (including Water) :	
	Grand Total:

Today's Date: No. of Calories

Breakfast:

_____

_____

_____

_____

_____

_____

_____

_____

_____

Lunch:

_____

_____

_____

_____

_____

_____

_____

_____

	No. of Calories
Dinner:	
Snacks & Beverages (including Water) :	
	Grand Total:

Today's Date:	No. of Calories
Breakfast:	
Lunch:	

No. of Calories

Dinner:

Snacks & Beverages (including Water) :

Grand Total:

Today's Date: | No. of Calories

Breakfast:

Lunch:

	No. of Calories
Dinner:	
Snacks & Beverages (including Water) :	
	Grand Total:

Today's Date:	No. of Calories
Breakfast:	
Lunch:	

	No. of Calories
Dinner:	
Snacks & Beverages (including Water):	
	Grand Total:

Today's Date: | No. of Calories

Breakfast:

Lunch:

	No. of Calories
Dinner:	
Snacks & Beverages (including Water) :	
	Grand Total:

Today's Date: | No. of Calories

Breakfast:

_____

_____

_____

_____

_____

_____

_____

_____

Lunch:

_____

_____

_____

_____

_____

_____

_____

_____

	No. of Calories
Dinner:	
Snacks & Beverages (including Water) :	
	Grand Total:

Today's Date: _____ | No. of Calories

Breakfast: _____

_____ | _____

_____ | _____

_____ | _____

_____ | _____

_____ | _____

_____ | _____

_____ | _____

_____ | _____

Lunch: _____

_____ | _____

_____ | _____

_____ | _____

_____ | _____

_____ | _____

_____ | _____

_____ | _____

_____ | _____

	No. of Calories
Dinner:	
Snacks & Beverages (including Water) :	
	Grand Total:

Today's Date:	No. of Calories
Breakfast:	
Lunch:	

	No. of Calories
Dinner:	
Snacks & Beverages (including Water) :	
	Grand Total:

Today's Date: | No. of Calories

Breakfast:

Lunch:

	No. of Calories
Dinner:	
Snacks & Beverages (including Water) :	
	Grand Total:

Today's Date: | No. of Calories

Breakfast:

Lunch:

	No. of Calories
Dinner:	
Snacks & Beverages (including Water) :	
	Grand Total:

Today's Date: No. of Calories

Breakfast:

Lunch:

	No. of Calories
Dinner:	
Snacks & Beverages (including Water) :	
	Grand Total:

Today's Date:	No. of Calories
Breakfast:	
Lunch:	

	No. of Calories
Dinner:	
Snacks & Beverages (including Water) :	
	Grand Total:

Today's Date: | No. of Calories

Breakfast:

Lunch:

	No. of Calories
Dinner:	
Snacks & Beverages (including Water) :	
	Grand Total:

Today's Date:	No. of Calories
Breakfast:	
Lunch:	

	No. of Calories
Dinner:	
Snacks & Beverages (including Water) :	
	Grand Total:

Today's Date: | No. of Calories

Breakfast:

Lunch:

	No. of Calories
Dinner:	
Snacks & Beverages (including Water) :	
	Grand Total:

Today's Date:	No. of Calories
Breakfast:	
Lunch:	

	No. of Calories
Dinner:	
Snacks & Beverages (including Water) :	
	Grand Total:

Today's Date: | No. of Calories

Breakfast:

Lunch:

	No. of Calories
Dinner:	
Snacks & Beverages (including Water) :	
	Grand Total:

Today's Date: | No. of Calories

Breakfast:

Lunch:

	No. of Calories
Dinner:	
Snacks & Beverages (including Water) :	
	Grand Total:

Today's Date: | No. of Calories

Breakfast:

Lunch:

	No. of Calories
Dinner:	
Snacks & Beverages (including Water) :	
	Grand Total:

Today's Date: | No. of Calories

Breakfast:

Lunch:

	No. of Calories
Dinner:	
Snacks & Beverages (including Water) :	
	Grand Total:

Today's Date: | No. of Calories

Breakfast:

Lunch:

	No. of Calories
Dinner:	
Snacks & Beverages (including Water) :	
	Grand Total:

Today's Date:	No. of Calories
Breakfast:	
Lunch:	

	No. of Calories
Dinner:	
Snacks & Beverages (including Water):	
	Grand Total:

Today's Date: | No. of Calories

Breakfast:

_____

Lunch:

	No. of Calories
Dinner:	
Snacks & Beverages (including Water) :	
	Grand Total:

Today's Date: | No. of Calories

Breakfast:

Lunch:

	No. of Calories
Dinner:	
Snacks & Beverages (including Water) :	
	Grand Total:

Today's Date: | No. of Calories

Breakfast:

Lunch:

	No. of Calories
Dinner:	
Snacks & Beverages (including Water) :	
	Grand Total:

Today's Date: | No. of Calories

Breakfast:

Lunch:

	No. of Calories
Dinner:	
Snacks & Beverages (including Water) :	
	Grand Total:

Today's Date: | No. of Calories

Breakfast:

Lunch:

	No. of Calories
Dinner:	
Snacks & Beverages (including Water):	
	Grand Total:

Today's Date: | No. of Calories

Breakfast:

Lunch:

	No. of Calories
Dinner:	
Snacks & Beverages (including Water) :	
	Grand Total:

Today's Date: | No. of Calories

Breakfast:

Lunch:

	No. of Calories
Dinner:	
Snacks & Beverages (including Water) :	
	Grand Total:

Today's Date: | No. of Calories

Breakfast:

Lunch:

No. of Calories

Dinner:

Snacks & Beverages (including Water) :

Grand Total:

Today's Date: _____ | No. of Calories

Breakfast: _____

_____ | _____

_____ | _____

_____ | _____

_____ | _____

_____ | _____

_____ | _____

_____ | _____

_____ | _____

Lunch: _____

_____ | _____

_____ | _____

_____ | _____

_____ | _____

_____ | _____

_____ | _____

_____ | _____

	No. of Calories
Dinner:	
Snacks & Beverages (including Water) :	
	Grand Total:

Today's Date:	No. of Calories
Breakfast:	
Lunch:	

	No. of Calories
Dinner:	
Snacks & Beverages (including Water) :	
	Grand Total:

Today's Date: | No. of Calories

Breakfast:

_____

_____

_____

_____

_____

_____

_____

_____

Lunch:

_____

_____

_____

_____

_____

_____

_____

_____

	No. of Calories
Dinner:	
Snacks & Beverages (including Water) :	
	Grand Total:

Today's Date:	No. of Calories
Breakfast:	
Lunch:	

	No. of Calories
Dinner:	
Snacks & Beverages (including Water) :	
	Grand Total:

Today's Date: | No. of Calories

Breakfast:

_____ | _____

_____ | _____

_____ | _____

_____ | _____

_____ | _____

_____ | _____

_____ | _____

_____ | _____

_____ | _____

Lunch:

_____ | _____

_____ | _____

_____ | _____

_____ | _____

_____ | _____

_____ | _____

_____ | _____

_____ | _____

	No. of Calories
Dinner:	
Snacks & Beverages (including Water) :	
	Grand Total:

Today's Date: | No. of Calories

Breakfast:

Lunch:

No. of Calories

Dinner:

_____

_____

_____

_____

_____

_____

_____

_____

Snacks & Beverages (including Water) :

_____

_____

_____

_____

_____

_____

_____

Grand Total:

_____

_____

Today's Date: | No. of Calories

Breakfast:

_____ | _____

_____ | _____

_____ | _____

_____ | _____

_____ | _____

_____ | _____

_____ | _____

_____ | _____

_____ | _____

Lunch:

_____ | _____

_____ | _____

_____ | _____

_____ | _____

_____ | _____

_____ | _____

_____ | _____

_____ | _____

	No. of Calories
Dinner:	
Snacks & Beverages (including Water) :	
	Grand Total:

Today's Date: | No. of Calories

Breakfast:

Lunch:

	No. of Calories
Dinner:	
Snacks & Beverages (including Water) :	
	Grand Total:

Today's Date: | No. of Calories

Breakfast:

Lunch:

	No. of Calories
Dinner:	
Snacks & Beverages (including Water) :	
	Grand Total:

Today's Date: | No. of Calories

Breakfast:

Lunch:

	No. of Calories
Dinner:	
Snacks & Beverages (including Water):	
	Grand Total:

Today's Date: | No. of Calories

Breakfast:

Lunch:

	No. of Calories
Dinner:	
Snacks & Beverages (including Water) :	
	Grand Total:

Today's Date:	No. of Calories
Breakfast:	
Lunch:	

No. of Calories

Dinner:

Snacks & Beverages (including Water) :

Grand Total:

Today's Date: | No. of Calories

Breakfast:

Lunch:

	No. of Calories
Dinner:	
Snacks & Beverages (including Water) :	
	Grand Total:

Today's Date:	No. of Calories
Breakfast:	
Lunch:	

	No. of Calories
Dinner:	
Snacks & Beverages (including Water) :	
	Grand Total:

Today's Date: | No. of Calories

Breakfast:

Lunch:

	No. of Calories
Dinner:	
Snacks & Beverages (including Water):	
	Grand Total:

Today's Date:	No. of Calories
Breakfast:	
Lunch:	

	No. of Calories
Dinner:	
Snacks & Beverages (including Water) :	
	Grand Total:

Today's Date: | No. of Calories

Breakfast:

Lunch:

	No. of Calories
Dinner:	
Snacks & Beverages (including Water) :	
	Grand Total:

Today's Date: | No. of Calories

Breakfast:

Lunch:

	No. of Calories
Dinner:	
Snacks & Beverages (including Water) :	
	Grand Total:

Today's Date: | No. of Calories

Breakfast:

_____

_____

_____

_____

_____

_____

_____

_____

Lunch:

_____

_____

_____

_____

_____

_____

_____

	No. of Calories
Dinner:	
Snacks & Beverages (including Water):	
	Grand Total:

Today's Date:	No. of Calories
Breakfast:	
Lunch:	

No. of Calories

Dinner:

Snacks & Beverages (including Water) :

Grand Total:

Today's Date: | No. of Calories

Breakfast:

_____

Lunch:

_____

	No. of Calories
Dinner:	
Snacks & Beverages (including Water):	
	Grand Total:

Today's Date:	No. of Calories
Breakfast:	
Lunch:	

	No. of Calories
Dinner:	
Snacks & Beverages (including Water) :	
	Grand Total:

Today's Date: | No. of Calories

Breakfast:

_____

_____

_____

_____

_____

_____

_____

_____

Lunch:

_____

_____

_____

_____

_____

_____

_____

	No. of Calories
Dinner:	
Snacks & Beverages (including Water) :	
	Grand Total:

Today's Date: | No. of Calories

Breakfast:

Lunch:

	No. of Calories
Dinner:	
Snacks & Beverages (including Water) :	
	Grand Total:

Today's Date:	No. of Calories
Breakfast:	
Lunch:	

No. of Calories

Dinner:

Snacks & Beverages (including Water) :

Grand Total:

Today's Date: | No. of Calories

Breakfast:

Lunch:

	No. of Calories
Dinner:	
Snacks & Beverages (including Water) :	
	Grand Total:

Today's Date:	No. of Calories
Breakfast:	
Lunch:	

	No. of Calories
Dinner:	
Snacks & Beverages (including Water) :	
	Grand Total:

Today's Date:	No. of Calories
Breakfast:	
Lunch:	

No. of Calories

Dinner:

Snacks & Beverages (including Water) :

Grand Total:

Today's Date: No. of Calories

Breakfast:

Lunch:

	No. of Calories
Dinner:	
Snacks & Beverages (including Water) :	
	Grand Total:

Today's Date: _____ | No. of Calories

Breakfast: _____ | _____

_____ | _____

_____ | _____

_____ | _____

_____ | _____

_____ | _____

_____ | _____

_____ | _____

_____ | _____

Lunch: _____ | _____

_____ | _____

_____ | _____

_____ | _____

_____ | _____

_____ | _____

_____ | _____

_____ | _____

_____ | _____

	No. of Calories
Dinner:	
Snacks & Beverages (including Water) :	
	Grand Total:

Today's Date: | No. of Calories

Breakfast:

Lunch:

	No. of Calories
Dinner:	
Snacks & Beverages (including Water):	
	Grand Total:

Today's Date: | No. of Calories

Breakfast:

Lunch:

	No. of Calories
Dinner:	
Snacks & Beverages (including Water) :	
	Grand Total:

Today's Date: | No. of Calories

Breakfast:

Lunch:

	No. of Calories
Dinner:	
Snacks & Beverages (including Water) :	
	Grand Total:

Today's Date:	No. of Calories
Breakfast:	
Lunch:	

No. of Calories

Dinner:

Snacks & Beverages (including Water) :

Grand Total:

Today's Date: | No. of Calories

Breakfast:

Lunch:

	No. of Calories
Dinner:	
Snacks & Beverages (including Water) :	
	Grand Total:

Today's Date:	No. of Calories
Breakfast:	
Lunch:	

	No. of Calories
Dinner:	
Snacks & Beverages (including Water) :	
	Grand Total:

Today's Date: | No. of Calories

Breakfast:

_____

Lunch:

	No. of Calories
Dinner:	
Snacks & Beverages (including Water) :	
	Grand Total:

Today's Date: | No. of Calories

Breakfast:

Lunch:

	No. of Calories
Dinner:	
Snacks & Beverages (including Water):	
	Grand Total:

Made in the USA
Las Vegas, NV
23 April 2022